The Rheumatoid Arthritis Diet:

Become Pain Free Forever with the Ultimate 30 Day Arthritis Cure Plan

Carl Preston

Table of Content

Introduction

Firstly, thank you for purchasing this eBook and secondly, I am sorry that you are suffering from arthritis or know someone who is. The good news is, this book has some great tips, recipes and instructions to dramatically improve your quality of life. You may think the road ahead of you is bleak, with too many painful obstacles to face but the truth is much more positive. There are lots of things you can do, starting today! 30 days from now, if you have taken the hints and tips on board, you will find yourself reaping the following benefits:

- You will lose excess weight
- You will have more energy
- Your joints won't feel as painful when you wake up
- You will be able to walk further distances
- You will be able move more freely
- Your stress levels will go down
- You will know how to use your mind to control your pain
- You won't need to take as many painkillers

Throughout this book, you are going to learn about ways in which you can work in harmony with your body using techniques of the mind, physical exercises and eating particular superfoods. Packed with instructions on how to implement new things into your daily schedule, you will be feeling your aches and pains fade away before you know it. As you turn each page, you will discover the foods that you can introduce into your diet that will specifically target inflammation in your joints. You will find how to stretch your muscles properly without causing injury and you will read guidance on using your mind as a natural pain reliever.

If you have read each of the points above and are eager to learn about how you can manage your arthritis and reduce the pain that you are feeling in just 30 days, and then make yourself comfortable, it's time for your new lease of life to start now!

Causes of Arthritis and How Your Diet Can Ease Your Pain

Arthritis is the name given for a pain in one or several parts of the body that has been caused by general wear and tear, a previous injury, obesity, infection, allergies, your genes, a physically demanding lifestyle or job and even food choices.

If you wake up each morning with a searing pain in your back or your joints are stiff, it is probably due to arthritis. So what's actually going on in the body? Well, we have connective tissue that helps to absorb shocks when we walk, run, or bang ourselves accidentally. Cartilage also allows us to move freely, which is great when we want to put our arms into a coat, reach high for something on a top shelf, type on a computer keyboard or play sports. Over time, the cartilage starts to break down which can be a result of an infection in the joints or it just happens with growing older.

There have been several scientific studies to show that diet can ease the symptoms of arthritis. Obesity is an obvious contributor to the worsening of arthritic symptoms, so weight loss will have a big impact on the reduction of pain. However, if you're not overweight, there are some foods you can avoid which will also help the intensity of pain to decrease.

Foods That Contribute to Reducing Arthritis Pains

Constant pain from arthritis can leave you feeling desperate to try anything, however the answer could be sitting in your kitchen right now. When you're feeling low because of your aching joints, it's easy to reach for the stodgy comfort food and the simple convenience food, but the trouble is the food you are eating could actually be contributing to your aches and causing more inflammation.

Whilst there are no foods, vitamins or minerals to cure arthritis, a change in diet can certainly help to reduce swelling, improve circulation and give you a boost in energy and vitality.

So what should you include in your diet?

- **Feast on fish**
    - Tuna
    - Mackerel
    - Herring
    - Salmon
    - Sardines

All of these types of oily fish are brimming with omega-3 fatty acids which are superb at fighting inflammation. If you can add two portions a week to your diet, you should start to feel your joints moving more easily.

- **It's Time To Get Oiled Up**
  - Avocado oil
  - Extra virgin olive oil
  - Safflower oil
  - Walnut oil
  - Coconut oil

Oils such as these are known to not only lower cholesterol but they also have similar properties to anti-inflammatory medication. They are also rich in omega-3 oils which will work hard at reducing inflammation.

- **Beautiful Berries**
  - Cherries
  - Strawberries
  - Blueberries
  - Raspberries
  - Blackberries

Purple berries are a great source of anthocyanin (try saying that without your teeth in!) which have been found to be responsible for improving cardiovascular health as well as reducing inflammation, so make yourself a yummy smoothie and ease your joints.

- **Ginger**
    - o Add a slice of ginger to a cup of tea or glass of lemonade
    - o Grate into cakes, biscuits, pancakes or curries
    - o Sprinkle ground ginger onto vegetables

Ginger is a fantastic antioxidant and has been used for centuries to treat a wide variety of ailments, including migraines, nausea, high blood pressure and the common cold however there is also evidence to support that sufferers of arthritis have seen a reduction in pain after regularly adding ginger to the diet.

- **Eat Your Greens (and whites!)**
    - o Broccoli
    - o Brussels Sprouts
    - o Cabbage
    - o Kale
    - o Cauliflower
    - o Bok Choy

Rather than eating to reduce pain, these cruciferous vegetables are more useful in preventing the onset of arthritis so if you don't already have this painful condition, you could take steps towards protecting yourself against it and if you do already have it, eating these vegetables should help to stop it developing in other parts of the body.

- **Vitamin C**
  - Oranges
  - Kiwi Fruit
  - Pineapple
  - Strawberries
  - Kidney Beans
  - Bell Peppers
  - Mangoes

According to an Oxford Journal, in 1997, 152 people with rheumatoid arthritis were studied and encouraged to increase their vitamin C intake. There were significant effects in the subjects and it was concluded that an increased intake of vitamin C resulted in less inflammation and pain.

- **Glucosamine Sulphate**
  - Used as a dietary supplement in liquid or tablet form

This chemical occurs naturally in the body and is used to build cartilage, fluid around the joints, ligaments and tendons. Ideal for sufferers of arthritis, particularly those who have pain located in their knees, hips or spine. It must be added that relief is not immediate and you do need to take at frequent intervals over a period of several weeks to feel the full benefits.

- **Vitamin D**
  - Bread
  - Yoghurt
  - Milk
  - Cheese

Be cautious with the dairy choices though as it can be connected to inflammation, which will have the opposite desired effect on your arthritis. It may be better to take a short stroll in some sunlight as an alternative.

- **Soybeans**
  - Try tofu or soy milk

If you can't stomach the thought of eating fish or you have allergies, soybeans are a brilliant alternative. As well as showing signs of reducing the painful symptoms of arthritis, they are also low in fat, high in fibre and protein and have all of the benefits of omega-3 fatty acids. These are a great choice if you're also trying to manage your weight.

- **Nuts and Seeds**
  - Brazil nuts
  - Walnuts
  - Pumpkin Seeds
  - Flaxseed

Added to cereal, yoghurts, salads or whatever you fancy, these little crunchy characters are perfect for preventing arthritis. The selenium found in the Brazil nuts is great at preventing knee pain and the fatty acids found in walnuts, pumpkin seed and flaxseed will reduce the need for visits to the doctor.

- **Green Tea**

Drink 3-4 cups of this a day and you should soon start to notice a difference in your pain levels. It is also a fantastic antioxidant so you will start to feel more energised too.

- **Quercetin – not just a great Scrabble word!**
    - Apples
    - Kale
    - Cherry Tomatoes
    - Onions
    - Leeks

Another antioxidant which works in a similar way to anti-inflammatories such as ibuprofen and aspirin.

- **Cherry Juice**

Recently, a study was carried our by the Arthritis and Rheumatism Journal which compared two groups of people with arthritis. Each group was given a bottle of juice to drink every day for six weeks. One bottle contained a placebo and the other contained the juice of around 50 tart cherries. The group who drank the cherry juice reported decreased pain compared to the group that had the placebo.

Healthy Habits That Reduce Arthritis

It is probably safe to say that the reason you have purchased this e-book is to find out how you can help yourself to reduce your pain caused by arthritis. So far we have looked at diet, but in addition to the super qualities of food, there are also some activities that you can do to ease your pain.

One thing to remember though, please don't do too much. If you push yourself to do more and more, it can increase the risk of injuring your joints rather than helping them. Find the right balance for your body, do enough to keep yourself mobile but not so much that the following few days mean you are bed bound because you are sore from too much exercise. Make sure you do plenty of stretching before you begin any exercise.

Get Your Groove On and Move

Whilst it may be tempting to lounge around in your pyjamas all day, barely moving from the sofa, you could actually be doing yourself more harm than good. You'll notice that when you wake first thing in the morning, your body is stiff and you'll experience pain in your joints. This is because you have stayed in a similar position for a long period of time.

It may hurt at first, but you will find your pain is eased and your joints feel suppler if you actually make an effort to move around more. This is not a suggestion to go hiking up a mountain for several hours but perhaps you could play your favourite music and swing your hips to the tune a couple of times a day?

If you have a dog, take it for a short walk three times a day, not only will the fresh air do you both good, the exercise is brilliant for you. Day by day you can increase the distance you walk too. Even if you don't have a dog, set yourself goals, on the first day just walk to the end of the street and back. The following day, increase the distance to the next visible lamppost and keep doing that until you're walking for at least an hour a day. If you have balancing struggles, you can purchase a couple of walking poles to give you that extra reassurance.

Take the Plunge

If you have a local swimming pool, swimming is an excellent way to exercise pain free. You may even find that there are groups or classes that you can join specifically for your age group, so it is worth taking a trip to a nearby leisure centre to find out what they offer. Studies have shown that people who take part in two half hour sessions in a warm pool each week will see an improvement in their range of movement and tenderness in their joints. A session can be anything you like, swimming lengths, water aerobics or simply treading water and chatting to a friend at the same time. The warmth of the water and the moving of joints whilst the water supports your weight will do wonders for you.

It's all about the Stretching

We are constantly told that it is important to take a break from screens which is why we have coffee breaks. We know it is good for us to get up and move around, but what we should also be doing is stretching several times a day. There are key areas in the body which should be stretched frequently throughout the day. These areas are the calves, thighs, hips, back, fingers, wrists, thumbs and back.

Calves

You should hold a stretch for approximately 30 seconds. To stretch your calves, lock your arms straight in front of you and place your hands against a wall or the back of a chair. Place one foot behind the other as though you're taking a large step and slowly bend your knee of the front leg, keeping the back leg straight. When you feel the calf stretch, hold for 30 seconds. Repeat with the other leg in front.

Thighs

To stretch your thigh, stay in the same position as above but bend both knees so that your front thigh is parallel to the floor. Lower yourself until you feel your thigh stretch. You can also stand straight and pull the heel of your foot to your bottom to stretch your thighs.

Hips

Cross your left foot in front of the right whilst standing beside a wall to your right. Hold your arm over your head, reaching toward the right side and you will feel a stretch along your left side. Repeat facing the other way with the right foot in front of the left and reaching toward the left. Hold each stretch for 30 seconds.

Back

Get on the floor on all fours. Stretch one leg out behind you and point your foot toward your head. Push your head backwards toward your foot. Repeat with the other leg. Hold each time for 30 seconds.

Yoga

A great way to improve flexibility is to practice regular yoga. Initially you may feel a bit silly standing with your arms in the air and lifting one foot off the floor, but I am sure that if you are fed up of being in pain, you are more than willing to give anything a try. Recent studies have shown that patients reported reduced tenderness in joints and a wider range of motion after taking part in yoga classes for a few weeks. Yoga is also a fantastic way to calm and relax yourself as well as socialise with other people.

Controlling Pain Using The Mind

You may think that by asking you to relax when your pain is at its worst is like asking you to put chocolate in your mouth without letting it melt. However, with practice, you will discover that relaxation techniques are superb for learning how to control your pain. So here's how to do it:

Step 1   Get yourself nice and comfy in a darkened room, preferably in a reclined position. You can choose to close your eyes or pick something in the room or on the ceiling to use as a focal point.

Step 2   Concentrate on your breathing. Consciously slow down your breaths and breathe deeper than you do normally. It helps if you repeat the word 'Relax' or 'Calm' in your mind as you breathe in and out.

After about three minutes of slowing down your breathing, you can introduce more ways of reaching a deeper relaxation specifically designed to reduce pain.

Step 3   Use any of the imagery techniques outlined here to see a notable difference in your pain levels.

(a) Imagine a needle being inserted into the area where you are feeling the most pain. Imagine a solution being injected through the needle into your body which has a numbing effect on the pain. You can imagine the cool solution spreading under your skin and around the affected area.

(b) Imagine the part of your body that is hurting is no longer part of you. Imagine it has temporarily been removed and is sitting in another part of the room, or even the house. Tell yourself that because your knee, wrist, back etc is sitting elsewhere, you can no longer feel the pain.

(c) Choose a part of the body to focus on which is not painful. Imagine it is getting warmer. Feel the sensation in your chosen part of the body that is getting warm and you will find that whilst you are concentrating on other parts of the body, your attention is taken away from the part of the body that is causing you pain.

(d) Use a trip down Memory Lane to remember a time when you were pain free or have fun imagining yourself in the future with zero pain. Tell yourself that this image is the truth and you are unable to feel pain anymore. Remember what is was like to be pain free and keep yourself focused on that thought.

(e) Counting sheep isn't just for sleep. You can decide what you would like to count either in your head or in the room. It could be tiny squares on the carpet or a pattern on the curtain or bees flying into a hive in your mind. Whatever you choose, count through the most painful episodes as a way of coping with the pain until the pain subsides.

(f) Give your pain a symbolic image that you find irritating. You could imagine that your chronic pain is an old, smelly person sitting next to you just won't stop talking. Imagine that you are making the old person smell lovely and clean and you are turning down the volume of their voice. They are getting quieter and quieter until eventually you can't hear them at all. You could also choose to turn your pain into a very bright light which is annoying you. As time passes by, you can dim the light which means you are dimming your pain.

It is completely up to you how long you would like to stay in a relaxed state for. Initially, it is probably advisable to aim for three 30 minute sessions each week and then once you are more comfortable with the techniques, you find that your abilities become stronger and you are able to stay in a relaxed state for longer periods.

Once you have practiced the above techniques frequently, you will find that you are able to achieve pain free results much more quickly. You will be able to reach a relaxed state within a few deep breaths instead of a few minutes of focussing on your breathing. Once you are experienced, you will have a greater sense of control over your pain and you will finally feel that you are able to cope.

Four Week Diet and Pain Reducing Plan

Week One

On the first week, follow these few rules to get you started on your journey to improved pain management, relaxation and possibly weight loss too. If you don't want to lose weight, just eat as you normally would but include some of the super foods mentioned earlier in this book.

A typical day to include anti-inflammatory foods can look like this:

> **Breakfast** – Spinach and Mushroom Frittata. This easy and satisfying breakfast is packed with nutrients known for their excellent ability at fighting inflammation.
>
> Don't forget to finish off with a lovely cup of Green Tea!
>
> Method – Sauté mushrooms, onion and a little garlic. Add spinach and ¼ cup water until the spinach wilts. Beat 6 large eggs with turmeric, salt and pepper and pour over the spinach and mushrooms and then transfer to the oven for 25-30 minutes until set in the middle and enjoy!
>
> **Lunch** – A simple lentil soup followed by an apple.
>
> Method - Finely chop onion, carrot, celery and garlic, cook until softened and then add ¾ cup of lentils and 14.5 ounces of low sodium chicken broth or vegetable soup. Cook on a low heat until soup thickens – about 6 minutes. Season to your liking.
>
> **Dinner** – Steamed Salmon with Greens
>
> Method – Simply season a fillet of salmon with salt and pepper and fold it in foil. Place in the oven for about 25 minutes and serve with your favourite green vegetables – delicious.

In your first week, it's probably best not to jump in at the deep end and take on too much so for now, just concentrate on stretching exercises as mentioned earlier to prepare your body for an increase in activity in the next few weeks.

Be sure to choose a time to do your stretches when you can give it your full attention. If you know that mornings are spent rushing around trying to get out of the house in time, then don't try to squeeze in ten minutes of stretching too because you will either end up rushing them or not doing them at all, with a promise to yourself to try again tomorrow, and as we know, tomorrow never comes! Choose a time to suit you when you can devote your time and energy into getting the positions right and your body will thank you for it more and more each day.

Reward yourself with a large glass of inflammation-reducing cherry juice and pat yourself on your back for taking some large leaps towards easing your pain.

Week 2

There's a huge variety of foods which have shown signs of easing the symptoms of arthritis – both osteoarthritis and rheumatoid arthritis. In particular, there has been plenty of research which suggests that introducing oily fish into your diet is beneficial for reducing inflammation in the joints. Why take cod liver oil supplements when you can create some superb tasting dishes? Boasting all the benefits of omega-3, you'll be able to tantalise your taste buds while enjoying improved mobility in your joints – it's a win-win!

Breakfast – Kippers

Kippers are a traditional way of serving smoked herring for breakfast, and have been popular for centuries across northern Europe. Every country has its favourite method, but for something a little different you can try poaching the kipper in an infusion of milk, red onion and a bay leaf for flavouring. Simply bring the pan up to a simmer and leave for a few minutes. Delicious!

Lunch – Mackerel on toast with horseradish

Simply mix some horseradish with a helping of crème fraiche and mustard powder, and set to one side. Fry off a couple of mackerel fillets skin side down for approximately 5 minutes, then give it another minute on the reverse side, following a generous seasoning of salt and pepper. Serve the hot mackerel with the horseradish mix, and a side salad of cucumber.

Dinner – Roasted trout with salsa

Not only is this dish packed full of flavour, with plenty of omega-3 fats to alleviate some of the pain that arthritis can cause, but it's a show-stopping gala meal which is ideal for entertaining guests. A specialist diet doesn't have to be boring!

You begin with a whole trout, cleaned and gutted (your fishmonger will be more than happy to do this for you). Place the trout into a large roasting tray together with a few halved lemons and par boiled potatoes. Spoon over a pureed mix of shallot, anchovy, mustard and a selection of herbs, drizzle with olive oil and roast in a hot oven for around 20 minutes. Serve with some roasted new potatoes, and you've got a healthy oily fish meal which is fit for a king!

Too much fish in one day could be a little over-powering, so feel free to mix and match your oily fish meals to create a more balanced diet over the week, however evidence suggests that the more portions you can introduce, the better you'll feel!

Now that you've got used to stretching on a daily basis, it's time to choose a form of exercise that you are happy to add into your weekly routine. Ideally, you will exercise a minimum of three times a week. Some people choose to do the same activity three times and others prefer to have a variety of activities and possibly by taking part in several pursuits over the course of the month. It is all down to your personal preference because you are more likely to succeed if you're doing something you enjoy. If you hate having to get dry and dressed in a tiny cubicle then swimming won't suit you but if you love the feeling of weightlessness in the water and the pressure off your joints, then you may be happy to endure a few minutes each week in a changing room.

So, this week, make sure you spend half an hour, three times a week doing one or more activities that has been mentioned previously, such as walking, swimming or yoga. If you are struggling to get up to half an hour initially then just do what you can. Whether you manage a minute or an hour, your efforts will pay off. An added bonus is that with all that extra movement, your body will tone up and your clothes will fit you better, they might even become too big – now there's a good problem to have!

Week 3

The Mediterranean basin which includes Greece and southern Italy contains some of the lowest percentages of arthritis-afflicted people in the world – and when you look at their diet, it's no coincidence. With very little red meat, relatively little dairy produce and an abundance of seafood and fresh vegetables, there's much we can adopt into our diet plan.

The traditional diet of the Mediterranean has not only been proven to aid with its anti-inflammatory properties, but has been shown to do a great deal to combat cardiovascular disease, diabetes and even a range of cancers. Reducing pain and stiffness and tasting great? Let's get started!

Breakfast – Muesli and fresh orange juice

Dieticians are nuts about...nuts. By mixing a broad range of nuts and seeds into a filling and nutritious breakfast muesli, you'll be introducing omega-3 fats, fibre and protein into your system for the most important meal of the day. Couple your muesli with a refreshing glass of orange juice, a fantastic dietary source of Vitamin C – which has been linked to a 30% reduced risk of developing rheumatoid arthritis.

Lunch – Greek salad

The more colours and varieties of vegetables you can cram into your Greek-style salad, the better. Your core ingredients would be lettuce, cucumber and sliced olives – with the salty hit of feta cheese cubes, although dairy has been suggested to be less than helpful for sufferers of arthritis. But the vital part – making your own dressing. By combining three parts olive oil to lemon juice, you'll save money and incorporate one of the healthiest oils around into your diet. Easy!

Dinner - Balsamic Chicken

This really simple dish takes only five minutes to prepare and 16 minutes to cook, so it's great for those with a busy lifestyle or someone who struggles to stand and cook for long periods of time. You will need two chicken breasts cut in half, chicken broth, lemon pepper seasoning, extra virgin olive oil, balsamic vinegar, garlic cloves, butter, parsley and cherry tomatoes.

Pound the chicken to 1/4inch. Sprinkle lemon pepper seasoning to both sides. Heat the oil and add the chicken. Cook for 7 minutes, turning once. Remove from the heat but keep warm. Mix together broth, garlic and vinegar and add to the frying pan for a few minutes until syrupy. Add butter, stir to melt. Pour over the chicken and garnish with parsley and cherry tomatoes.

Now that you're in your third week, you will have been stretching every day for two weeks and exercising for a week, by now you will already start to see improvements in your fitness levels and increased mobility in your joints. This week you can revisit your youth and crank up the volume on your favourite tunes. Before you know it you will be dancing around the kitchen and singing into your mop. On top of that, you'll be loosening up your stiff joints, increasing your heart rate and boosting your serotonin levels. Happy days!

Week 4

You've now completed almost a month of your new regime yet there are still lots of great combinations are foods for you to try and by now you should have a good idea of the things that have been working best for your body. Below, you'll find another great sample meal plan containing key ingredients to regain some control over your arthritis.

Breakfast – Raspberry Green Tea Smoothie

This is a fantastic on-the-go breakfast which can make ahead of time and take with you to drink in the car or on public transport on your way to work. You will need some chilled green tea, frozen strawberries, a banana, honey (preferably manuka honey for even more added benefits due to its antibiotic type qualities) and protein powder. Throw all the ingredients into a blender until smooth and then pour over ice and drink or transfer to a bottle to take with you. Perfect.

Lunch – Sweet Potato Soup

With sweet potatoes, ginger, orange juice and olive oil, this soup packs a powerful punch to knock inflammation right where it hurts. You can even double or triple the quantity to freeze as this soup can really stand the test of time. Great if you need something quick and easy to take to work, especially if you have use of a microwave. Your colleagues will be transfixed by the tempting aroma that wafts around the kitchen or staff room. You can place bets with yourself on how many times you're going to get asked for the recipe. Speaking of which...

You will need sweet potatoes, extra virgin olive oil, kosher salt, cracked pepper, thinly sliced leeks or onions, 1 inch piece of fresh ginger, peeled and minced, minced garlic, dry white wine, vegetable broth, orange juice and fresh thyme leaves.

Cut the sweet potato into chunks and roast for about 45 minutes. Grab a huge cooking pot and cook the onions or leaks for about 8 minutes then add in the garlic and ginger. Add the wine and bring to the boil. Cook until the wine has reduced (evaporated) and then add the broth. Stir in the roasted sweet potatoes and thyme before cooking for a further 20 minutes. Puree the soup using a blender. All done!

Dinner – Quinoa and Turkey Stuffed Peppers

Arthritis enemies come in the form on many things, some of which are red peppers, turkey and olive oil, so let's throw them all together and see what we get!

You will need uncooked quinoa, water, salt, turkey sausage, chicken stock, extra virgin olive oil, pecans, fresh herbs and three bell peppers.

Mix together the quinoa, water and salt and boil until all the water has been absorbed. Stir in the turkey sausage, chicken stock, olive oil and herbs. Remove all seeds from the peppers before cutting in half and boiling for 5 minutes. Fill each pepper with the quinoa mixture and bake in the oven for 15 minutes – delicious.

Now after three weeks of bouncing around, it's time you had a rest and did something less physical. That's right; you're going to use the power of the mind to block the pain signals that you are receiving. Take a look at the previous chapters for the full instruction on how find inner strength and abilities. Use the techniques mentioned previously to disengage the painful parts of your body or train yourself to dull the pain to a quiet muffle rather than having shout at you and control you every day.

So that brings us to the end of the sample meal plan and ideas of how to implement new activities into your life. There are plenty more recipes available so be sure to do some of your own research to really reach your true potential and turn your life around. The world is on your door step and all you have to do is take one step to reach it. Do it now!

Conclusion

By now you have either been implementing everything we have talked about over the course of a month or you have ready the book from cover to cover and you are itching to get started. The most important thing to remember is that you must do what feels right for you. Sometimes we get a little too giddy and we make all sorts of crazy statements about what we are going to do and how our lives will be transformed and then when it actually comes down to it, we realise that we were a little too ambitious and the goals we set ourselves were out of reach. When we bite off more than we can chew, we feel completely out of our comfort zones so we give up. We go back to our comfort zone and we feel guilty. We blame ourselves for failing to keep promises and this drives us to return to our old ways. In this case, old ways means more pain and more inflammation, so in a very literal sense, by failing to stick to these new ways of coping with your arthritis, the only person you will be hurting is yourself.

Many people get to the end of this book ready to do absolutely everything that is offered as advice all at once. People rush out to the supermarket to buy every ingredient listed on these pages, they sign up for an annual gym membership and they draw up a schedule and stick it on the fridge which shows three hours each day is dedicated to walking, swimming and mind exercises.

Whilst it is great that this book is so inspiring, it is also important to remember that you must set yourself achievable goals. Goals that you know you can and will stick to because the longer you can commit to your new lifestyle, the more benefits you will see and the more likely you are to be able to change your life for the better forever.

Let me give you two examples. Bill and Margaret are both overweight and they both suffer from arthritis. Both of them read this book all the way through and are keen to implement the new ways that they have read about. Both of them are used to eating a full English breakfast each morning, watching daytime television until lunch time, drinking several cups of tea with full fat milk with a biscuit at regular intervals, enjoying homemade pie for lunch, pottering in the garden in the afternoon, with a few more cups of tea thrown in and then settling down to fish and chips in the evening with a lovely helping of apple pie. Now, because they have both read this book, they decided to make some changes, however they each have a different approach. Let's have a look at what they do.

Bill

In the first week Bill decides to still have a full English breakfast but he decides to change the oil he uses for frying to olive oil. He also swaps his morning cup of coffee to a glass of cherry juice. He watches an hour of television and then stands up and does a few stretches before putting on his favourite music and sings along whilst moving swiftly around the room. He is a little out of breath afterwards but he feels good. For lunch, he makes his usual slice of homemade pie but serves some broccoli with it and has some fruit as a dessert. In the afternoon he sits in his garden and tries some mind exercises for 10 minutes in the peace and quiet. Later on instead of battered fish and chips, Bill makes himself a fillet of salmon and chips which he thoroughly enjoys. Bill is looking forward to keeping up these few small changes. He goes to bed that night happy.

Margaret

In the first week, Margaret is keen to do everything she has read about in the book. Instead of having a full English breakfast, she has muesli with soy milk. She isn't too keen on the taste but she feels very healthy. Straight after breakfast, she walks to the local swimming pool and swims 20 lengths of the pool before walking back home. Her legs are aching and she is very hungry. She makes a salad with cheese and pumpkin seeds and afterwards finds herself ready for a nap so she sits in her chair and falls asleep for an hour. She wakes up feeling a little sore from the exercise earlier that day. She makes herself a cup of green tea and grates some ginger in to it even though she doesn't really like it and she only manages to drink half of it. Later on she is very hungry so has her usual fish and chips before trying some yoga but is too sore from earlier and gives up. Margaret has decided that these new ways to reduce arthritis are too difficult and she doesn't want to try it anymore. She goes to bed that night unhappy.

The above two examples are to show you how drastic changes to your lifestyle are not always a good thing and before long, you will start to crave your old ways, which means your goals of being pain free in a month may never be attained. If you take the advice on board, and do as Bill does and make small changes to your lifestyle, you won't feel like you are missing out on anything and you will be much more likely to stick to it.

Therefore, like Bill, you will soon find that you can live a healthier lifestyle and reduce your aches and pains.

To recap, the benefits of implementing some or all of the foods and exercises mentioned throughout the book are:

- Reduced inflammation in and around the joints
- Increased flexibility in your joints
- A smaller waistline
- More energy
- A better quality of life

Thank you for taking the time to read this book. You are now ready and armed to make some very important changes to your life; it's time for you to start living again. Enjoy!

Preview of "The Anti-Aging Superfoods Diet"

Introduction

This book is a comprehensive overview of a diet that will help you to maintain and prevent outward and inward aging. When you've completed this four week plan, your skin will be healthier, and your body will feel stronger, inside and out.

In this book, we will discover exactly what foods you need to make a part of your diet in order to help you become healthier, look younger, and have more energy. The four week plan is a perfect jumping-off point towards a healthier lifestyle and a younger you!

Soon you will be looking in the mirror and smiling at what you see in front of you. You will see a new glow to your skin, a sparkle in your eyes and a shine to your hair. We could all do with a bit of that couldn't we? As long as you are prepared to take on board the information inside this book and follow the advice given, there is no reason why you won't see an improvement in your energy levels and your appearance.

The best bit is, you don't have to stop after just four weeks. The guidance you are about to read will teach you how you can alter your current lifestyle on a more permanent basis, if you wish.

Your body is yours to do what you like with so if you have a particular goal in mind and only want to follow the information for a short period of time, you can! If you would rather see continuous improvement and reverse your aging from now until forever more, you can do that too!

So what will be covered in this book? Well, let me tell you!

- **Chapter One** – here we see the connection between diet and aging and how your lifestyle can actually speed up the aging process depending on what you allow into your system. You will learn how you may have been stalling weight loss and depleting energy levels and you will find out how to turn this information into a long term plan to **reach and maintain your goals.**

- **Chapter Two** – this chapter is about my favourite thing, food! You'll find out what foods can **boost your immunity** and **flush out toxins** but don't worry, there isn't a cardboard flavoured cracker in sight! All the foods we talk about are **naturally delicious** as well as helpful for giving you **a body to be proud of.**

- **Chapter Three** – Want to **jog for 10 miles without getting breathless**? Go on then! This chapter explores how your diet can change you from being a slob on the sofa to an athletic Adonis! I kid you not! Read this chapter for tips on which foods to eat to not only get you through the normal working day but to also allow you to spend your evenings and early mornings getting fit too!

- **Chapter Four** – Probably the most popular chapter – here we explore how you can **melt away the pounds** just by making different choices about the types of food that you put on your plate. Learn how to **block cravings** and how to **feel satisfied for longer**.

- **Chapters 5-8** – The **Step By Step Guide**. Some people like to read a summary of facts and then carve their own path and others prefer to have a strict set of rules to follow. The beauty of this book is that it can do both. If you like instructions, these chapters are perfect for you. Hints and tips will guide you through four weeks so that by the end, you will see results but not only that, you will have learned all the tools you need to continue your successes if you wish.

- **Chapter 9** – If you're a little afraid of the long term journey, this chapter will give you all the reassurance that you need to keep going. You will have seen **fantastic progress** so far and will no doubt be motivated to continue. You'll be hearing **positive comments** from friends and family and you'll **feel fitter** than you ever have.

So now that you have seen what awaits you in each of these chapters, go and make yourself a drink, find a comfortable position and start reading this book. This is the first day of the rest of your fit and healthy life – enjoy!

Table of contents

Chapter 1: The Basics

The Connection between Diet and Aging:

Your skin is a window to your overall health. It is, after all, your body's largest organ. The way your skin looks can tell you a lot about the health of your body. There are two kinds of aging, but only one kind do we have any control over. **Extrinsic** aging is the effect of environmental factors on your skin, such as pollution, smoking, sun exposure, sleep deprivation and, last but not least, improper nutrition. Your skin is the largest organ in your body; it will reflect what you look like on the inside.

Losing Weight:

What many people do not know is that when a person is overweight, or when their blood sugar levels are elevated, a biochemical reaction begins that breaks down the structure of their skin. When you combine high blood sugar and extra pounds with environmental factors, you have a recipe for the deterioration of your skin.

The best way to tackle this problem is from the inside, out! If your body is healthy, your skin is healthy and you will *look* healthy!

Higher Energy Level:

It's no secret that how we eat affects how much energy we have. Loading up on carbohydrates and refined sugar provides a short term boost followed by a hard crash. When our energy crashes, we crave something to boost it immediately, which usually ends up being more carbs or sugar. It's a vicious cycle that is difficult to break. However, if you start thinking about your long-term energy needs, and eat accordingly, you will find your need for that immediate "high" diminishing.

Long Term Plan:

While this diet is a great crash-course in detoxing and healthy eating, it is not enough by itself! If you want to feel and look younger, you will have to make lifestyle changes that stick around longer than the four week diet. Commit! Now is the time to do it. Don't wait for New Years to make the change. Don't wait for that check-up with your doctor where you get "bad news." Do it today!

Chapter 2: Foods to Prevent and Slow Down Aging

Your skin is a mirror to your health. Proper nutrition will aid you in becoming healthier and that health will be reflected in your skin and appearance. Compiled here is a list of foods that will slow down aging.

Fruits

Berries:

Blackberries, blueberries, strawberries and plums are all very high in antioxidants. Antioxidants are nutrients and enzymes that your body needs to repair and prevent damage to your body tissues.

Red Grapes:

Resveratrol is an antioxidant found in red grapes. Antioxidants fight free radicals that contribute to cell deterioration. This includes your skin cells, so these antioxidants are crucial to maintaining healthy, young looking skin.

Kiwi:

Delicious, sweet kiwi are high in Vitamin C and E. Making kiwi a part of your diet can add firmness to your skin and slow down the process of the formation of fine lines.

Pomegranate:

Pomegranates are a true superfood. Rich in riboflavin and phosphorus, eating pomegranates regularly can increase your body's production of collagen.

Vegetables

Tomatoes:

Tomatoes contain lycopene, an antioxidant that combats free radicals, harmful molecules or ions that damage healthy cells, including skin cells. Eating tomatoes can prevent these free radicals from deteriorating your cells.

Eggplant:

The beautiful purple peal of eggplant contains *nasunin*, another antioxidant that battles harmful free radicals. Studies have also shown that *nasunin* can help prevent or slow down Alzheimer's disease.

Grains

Oats, Quinoa, Barley, Wheat, and Brown Rice: All whole grains can play a positive role in looking and feeling younger. Whole grains are crucial to keeping your blood vessels healthy, which means less spider veins or varicose veins.

Protein

Salmon:

Salmon contains something called "fatty acids." Fatty acids, such as omega-3, are vital to the health of your cell membranes. The cell membrane is responsible for keeping bad things out, and promoting the passage of good nutrients throughout your body. These cell membranes are also responsible for holding in water, which means healthier, plumper skin.

Free Books

Do not miss my temporary offers on http://bit.ly/FreeChangeBooks.

These offers are temporary and it might take days or only hours until they expire. Do not let it happen and snap up the existing offers while they last!

Check Out My Other Books

Here you will find a detailed description of my other books with a link to their Amazon page where you can acquire them and enjoy them while you learn excellent tips and advice on Health, Dieting, Relaxation techniques and much more!

The Ultimate Headache-Free Migraine Diet:

A Comprehensive 30 Day Migraine Cure Plan.

http://bit.ly/ChangeMigraineCure

The Zen Gardens Stress Cure:

Four Seasons of Relaxation Techniques and Zen Mindfulness

http://bit.ly/ZenChangeBook

The Rheumatoid Arthritis Diet:

Become Pain Free Forever with the Ultimate 30 Day Arthritis Cure Plan

http://bit.ly/ArthritisChangeBook

Real Meditation:

An Alternative Approach to Meditation Techniques to Achieve Inner Peace

http://bit.ly/ChangeRealMeditation

Made in the USA
Lexington, KY
07 July 2016